WHAT DOES EATING

PLANT-BASED MEAN?

A Cookbook That Prevents Obesity and Diabetes

The Green Solution

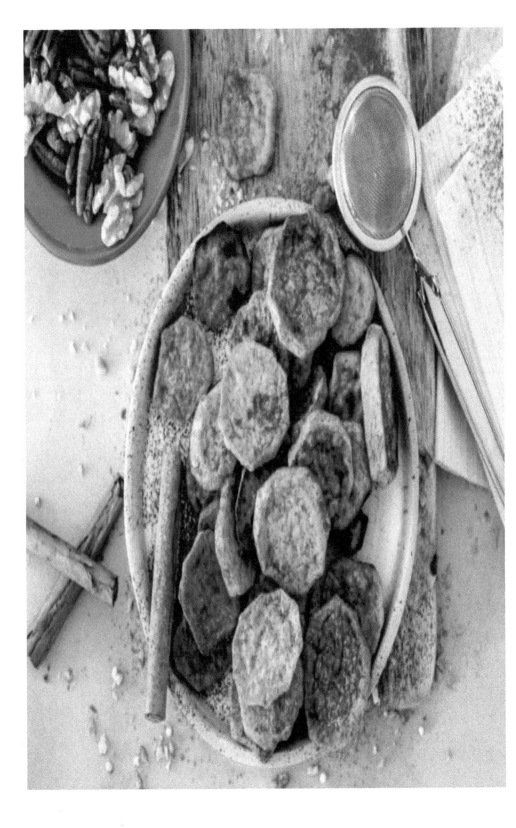

Table of Contents

INTRODUCTION

A plant-based diet is a diet consisting mostly or entirely of plant-based foods with no animal products or artificial ingredients. While a plant-based diet avoids or has limited animal products, it is not necessarily vegan. This includes not only fruits and vegetables, but also nuts, seeds, oils, whole grains, legumes, and beans. It doesn't mean that you are vegetarian or vegan and never eat meat, eggs, or dairy.

Vegetarian diets have also been shown to support health, including a lower risk of developing coronary heart disease, high blood pressure, diabetes, and increased longevity.

Plant-based diets offer all the necessary carbohydrates, vitamins, protein, fats, and minerals for optimal health, and are often higher in fiber and phytonutrients. However, some vegans may need to add a supplement to ensure they receive all the nutrients required.

Who says that plant-based diets are limited or boring? There are lots of delicious recipes that you can use to make mouthwatering, healthy, plant-based dishes that will satisfy your cravings. If you're eating these plant-based foods regularly, you can maintain a healthy weight without obsessing about calories and avoid diseases that result from bad dietary habits.

Benefits of a Plant-Based Diet

Eating a plant-based diet improves the health of your gut so you are better able to absorb the nutrients from food that support your immune system and reduce inflammation. Fiber can lower cholesterol and stabilize blood sugar, and it's great for good bowel management.

- **A Plant-Based Diet May Lower Your Blood Pressure**
  High blood pressure, or hypertension, can increase the risk for health issues, including heart disease, stroke, and type 2 diabetes and reduce blood pressure and other risky conditions.

- **A Plant-Based Diet May Keep Your Heart Healthy**
  Saturated fat in meat can contribute to heart issues when eaten in excess, so plant-based foods can help keep your heart healthy.

- **A Plant-Based Diet May Help Prevent Type 2 Diabetes**
  Animal foods can increase cholesterol levels, so eating a plant-based diet filled with high-quality plant foods can reduce the risk of developing type 2 diabetes by 34 percent.

- **Eating a Plant-Based Diet Could Help You Lose Weight**
  Cutting back on meat can help you to maintain a healthy weight because a plant-based diet is naturally satisfying and rich in fiber.

- **Following a Plant-Based Diet Long Term May Help You Live Longer**
  If you stick with healthy plant-based foods your whole body will be leaner and healthier, allowing you to stay healthy and vital as you age.

- **A Plant-Based Diet May Decrease Your Risk of Cancer**
  Vegetarians have an 18 percent lower risk of cancer compared to non-vegetarians. This is because a plant-based diet is rich of fibers and healthy nutrients.

- **A Plant-Based Diet May Improve Your Cholesterol**
  High cholesterol can lead to fatty deposits in the blood, which can restrict blood flow and potentially lead to heart attack, stroke, heart disease, and many other problems. A plant-based diet can help in maintaining healthy cholesterol levels.

- **Ramping Up Your Plant Intake May Keep Your Brain Strong**
  Increased consumption of fruits and vegetables is associated with a 20 percent reduction in the risk of cognitive impairment and dementia. So plant foods can help protect your brain from multiple issues.

What to Eat in Plant-Based Diets

Fruits: Berries, citrus fruits, pears, peaches, pineapple, bananas, etc.

Vegetables: Kale, spinach, tomatoes, broccoli, cauliflower, carrots, asparagus, peppers, etc.

Starchy vegetables: Potatoes, sweet potatoes, butternut squash, etc.

Whole grains: Brown rice, rolled oats, farro, quinoa, brown rice pasta, barley, etc.

Healthy fats: Avocados, olive oil, coconut oil, unsweetened coconut, etc.

Legumes: Peas, chickpeas, lentils, peanuts, black beans, etc.

Seeds, nuts, and nut butters: Almonds, cashews, macadamia nuts, pumpkin seeds, sunflower seeds, natural peanut butter, tahini, etc.

Unsweetened plant-based milks: Coconut milk, almond milk, cashew milk, etc.

Spices, herbs, and seasonings: Basil, rosemary, turmeric, curry, black pepper, salt, etc.

Condiments: Salsa, mustard, nutritional yeast, soy sauce, vinegar, lemon juice, etc.

Plant-based protein: Tofu, tempeh, plant-based protein sources or powders with no added sugar or artificial ingredients.

Beverages: Coffee, tea, sparkling water, etc.

What Not to Eat in Plant-Based Diets

Fast food: French fries, cheeseburgers, hot dogs, chicken nuggets, etc.

Added sugars and sweets: Table sugar, soda, juice, pastries, cookies, candy, sweet tea, sugary cereals, etc.

Refined grains: White rice, white pasta, white bread, bagels, etc.

Packaged and convenience foods: Chips, crackers, cereal bars, frozen dinners, etc.

Processed vegan-friendly foods: Plant-based meats like; Tofurkey, faux cheeses, vegan butters, etc.

Artificial sweeteners: Equal, Splenda, Sweet'N Low, etc.

Processed animal products: Bacon, lunch meats, sausage, beef jerky, etc.

Day 1:

Breakfast (304 calories)

- 1 serving Berry-Kefir Smoothie

A.M. Snack (95 calories)

- 1 medium apple

Lunch (374 calories)

- 1 serving Green Salad with Pita Bread & Hummus

P.M. Snack (206 calories)

- 1/4 cup dry-roasted unsalted almonds

Dinner (509 calories)

- 1 serving Beefless Vegan Tacos
- 2 cups mixed greens
- 1 serving Citrus Vinaigrette

Day 2:

Breakfast (258 calories)

- 1 serving Cinnamon Roll Overnight Oats
- 1 medium orange

A.M. Snack (341 calories)

- 1 cup low-fat plain Greek yogurt
- 1 medium peach
- 3 Tbsps slivered almonds

Lunch (332 calories)

- 1 serving Thai-Style Chopped Salad with Sriracha Tofu

P.M. Snack (131 calories)

- 1 large pear

Dinner (458 calories)

- 1 serving Mexican Quinoa Salad

Day 3:

Breakfast (258 calories)

- 1 serving Cinnamon Roll Overnight Oats
- 1 medium orange

A.M. Snack (95 calories)

- 1 medium apple

Lunch (463 calories)

- 1 serving Thai-Style Chopped Salad with Sriracha Tofu
- 1 large pear

P.M. Snack (274 calories)

- 1/3 cup dried walnut halves
- 1 medium peach

Dinner (419 calories)

- 1 serving Eggs in Tomato Sauce with Chickpeas & Spinach
- 11-oz. slice whole-wheat baguette

SOUPS & SALADS

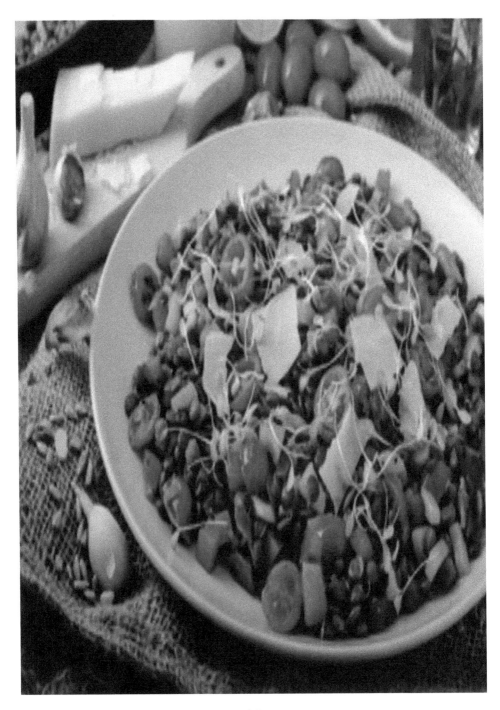

Servings: 10

Preparation Time: 20 minutes + chilling time

Per Serving: Calories: 349; Fat: 15.1g; Carbs: 40.9g; Protein: 15.4g

Ingredients:

- 4 cups arugula
- 4 cups Romaine lettuce, torn into pieces
- 6 tablespoons fresh lemon juice
- 3 cups green lentils, rinsed
- 2 cups baby spinach
- 1/4 cup oil-packed sun-dried tomatoes, rinsed and chopped
- Sea salt and ground black pepper, to taste
- 1/2 cup fresh basil, chopped
- 1 cup shallots, chopped
- 4 garlic cloves, finely chopped
- 10 tablespoons extra-virgin olive oil

Procedure:

1. Take a large-sized saucepan, bring 4 ½ cups of the water and red lentils to a boil.
2. Immediately turn the heat to a simmer and continue to cook your lentils for a further 15 to 17 minutes or until they've softened but not mushy.
3. Now, drain and let it cool completely.

4. Then, transfer the lentils to a salad bowl; toss the lentils with the remaining ingredients until well combined.
5. Finally, serve chilled or at room temperature.

Traditional Indian Chana Chaat Salad

Servings: 8

Preparation Time: 45 minutes + chilling time

Per Serving: Calories: 604; Fat: 23.1g; Carbs: 80g; Protein: 25.3g

Ingredients:

- 2 green chilies, seeded and thinly sliced
- 4 San Marzano tomatoes, diced
- 2 Persian cucumbers, sliced
- 2 onions, chopped
- 1 teaspoon Kashmiri chili powder
- 2 bell peppers, seeded and thinly sliced
- 2 pounds dry chickpeas, soaked overnight
- 4 handfuls of baby spinach
- 8 curry leaves, chopped
- 2 tablespoons chaat masala
- 4 tablespoons fresh lemon juice, or to taste
- 8 tablespoons olive oil
- 2 teaspoons agave syrup
- 4 tablespoons sesame seeds, lightly toasted
- 4 tablespoons fresh cilantro, roughly chopped
- 1 teaspoon coriander seeds
- 1 teaspoon mustard seeds

Procedure:

1. First, drain the chickpeas and transfer them to a large saucepan.
2. Cover the chickpeas with water by 2 inches and bring it to a boil.
3. Now, immediately turn the heat to a simmer and continue to cook for approximately 40 minutes.
4. Then, toss the chickpeas with the tomatoes, cucumber, onion, peppers, spinach, chili powder, curry leaves, and chaat masala.
5. Take a small mixing dish, thoroughly combine the lemon juice, olive oil, agave syrup, mustard seeds, and coriander seeds.
6. Finally, garnish with sesame seeds and fresh cilantro. Bon appétit!

Homemade Thai-Style Tempeh and Noodle Salad

Servings: 6

Preparation Time: 45 minutes

Per Serving: Calories: 494; Fat: 14.5g; Carbs: 75g; Protein: 18.7g

Ingredients:

- 12 ounces tempeh
- 8 tablespoons rice vinegar
- 8 tablespoons soy sauce
- 4 garlic cloves, minced
- 2 small-sized limes, freshly juiced
- 10 ounces rice noodles
- 2 carrots, julienned
- 2 shallots, chopped
- 6 handfuls Chinese cabbage, thinly sliced
- 6 handfuls kale, torn into pieces
- 2 bell peppers, seeded and thinly sliced
- 2 bird's eye chilies, minced
- 1/2 cup peanut butter
- 4 tablespoons agave syrup

Procedure:

1. First, place the tempeh, 2 tablespoons of the rice vinegar, soy sauce, garlic, and lime juice in a ceramic dish; let it marinate for about 40 minutes.
2. Meanwhile, cook the rice noodles according to the package directions.
3. Now, drain your noodles and transfer them to a salad bowl.
4. Then, add the carrot, shallot, cabbage, kale, and peppers to the salad bowl.
5. After that, add in the peanut butter, the remaining 2 tablespoons of the rice vinegar, and agave syrup and toss to combine well.
6. Lastly, top with the marinated tempeh and serve immediately. Enjoy!

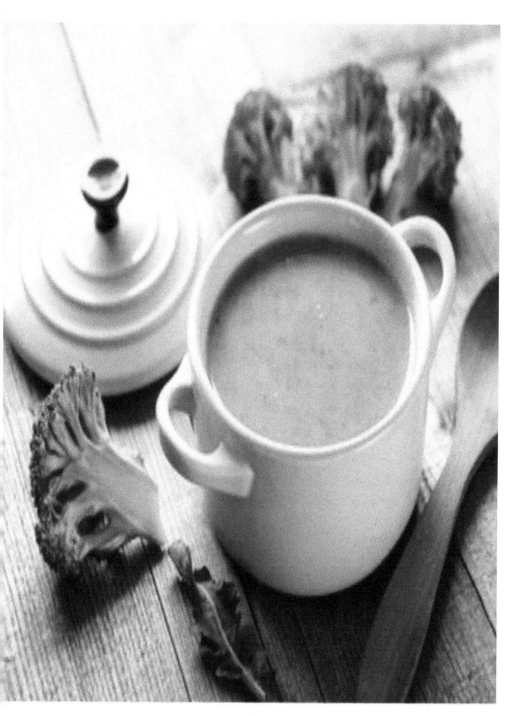

Servings: 8

Preparation Time: 35 minutes

Per Serving: Calories: 334; Fat: 24.5g; Carbs: 22.5g; Protein: 10.2g

Ingredients:

- 4 tablespoons olive oil
- 2 pounds broccoli florets
- 2 onions, chopped
- 2 celery ribs, chopped
- 2 parsnips, chopped
- 2 teaspoons garlic, chopped
- 6 cups vegetable broth
- 1 teaspoon dried dill
- 1 teaspoon dried oregano
- Sea salt and ground black pepper, to taste
- 4 tablespoons flaxseed meal
- 2 cups full-fat coconut milk

Procedure:

1. Take a heavy-bottomed pot, heat the olive oil over medium-high heat.
2. Now, sauté the broccoli onion, celery, and parsnip for about 5 minutes, stirring periodically.
3. Add in the garlic and continue sautéing for 1 minute or until fragrant.

4. Then, stir in the vegetable broth, dill, oregano, salt, and black pepper; bring to a boil.
5. Immediately reduce the heat to a simmer and let it cook for about 20 minutes.
6. Now, puree the soup using an immersion blender until creamy and uniform.
7. Return the pureed mixture to the pot.
8. Then, fold in the flaxseed meal and coconut milk; continue to simmer until heated through or about 5 minutes.
9. Lastly, ladle into four serving bowls and enjoy!

Servings: 8

Preparation Time: 20 minutes + chilling time

Per Serving: Calories: 418; Fat: 15g; Carbs: 62.9g; Protein: 12.4g

Ingredients:

- 2 cups red lentils, rinsed
- 2 large carrots, julienned
- 2 Persian cucumbers, thinly sliced
- 2 sweet onions, chopped
- 1 cups golden raisins
- 1/2 cup fresh mint, snipped
- 1/2 cup fresh basil, snipped
- 1/2 cup extra-virgin olive oil
- 1/2 cup lemon juice, freshly squeezed
- 2 teaspoons grated lemon peel
- 1 teaspoon fresh ginger root, peeled and minced
- 1 teaspoon granulated garlic
- 2 teaspoons ground allspice
- Sea salt and ground black pepper, to taste

Procedure:

1. Take a large-sized saucepan, bring 3 cups of the water and 1 cup of the lentils to a boil.
2. Immediately turn the heat to a simmer and continue to cook your lentils for a further 15 to 17

minutes or until they've softened but are not mushy yet.

3. Now, drain and let it cool completely.
4. Transfer the lentils to a salad bowl; add in the carrot, cucumber, and sweet onion.
5. Then, add the raisins, mint, and basil to your salad.
6. Take a small mixing dish, whisk the olive oil, lemon juice, lemon peel, ginger, granulated garlic, allspice, salt, and black pepper.
7. In the end, dress your salad and serve well-chilled. Bon appétit!

Servings: 10

Preparation Time: 10 minutes + chilling time

Per Serving: Calories: 198; Fat: 12.9g; Carbs: 17.5g; Protein: 5.5g

Ingredients:

- 2 chipotle peppers, seeded and chopped
- 1/2 cup fresh basil leaves, chopped
- 10 ounces canned chickpeas, drained and rinsed
- 1/2 cup fresh parsley leaves, chopped
- 4 tablespoons fresh mint leaves
- 2 Italian peppers, seeded and chopped
- 2,1/2 pounds asparagus, trimmed and cut into bite-sized pieces
- 4 tablespoons fresh chives, chopped
- 2 teaspoons garlic, minced
- 1/2 cup extra-virgin olive oil
- 2 tablespoons balsamic vinegar
- 2 tablespoons fresh lime juice
- 1/2 teaspoon ground cumin
- Sea salt and freshly cracked peppercorns, to taste
- 4 tablespoons soy sauce
- 1/2 teaspoon ground allspice

Procedure:

1. First, bring a large pot of salted water with the asparagus to a boil; let it cook for 2 minutes; drain and rinse.
2. Then, transfer the asparagus to a salad bowl.
3. Now, toss the asparagus with the chickpeas, peppers, herbs, garlic, olive oil, vinegar, lime juice, soy sauce, and spices.
4. Lastly, toss to combine and serve immediately. Bon appétit!

Servings: 8

Preparation Time: 10 minutes + chilling time

Per Serving: Calories: 240; Fat: 14.1g; Carbs: 29g; Protein: 4.4g

Ingredients:

- 2 teaspoons garlic, minced
- 2 Persian cucumbers, sliced
- 4 cups grape tomatoes, halved
- 1/2 teaspoon dried thyme
- 3 pounds green beans, trimmed
- 1/2 cup olive oil
- 2 teaspoons deli mustard
- Sea salt and ground black pepper, to taste
- 4 tablespoons tamari sauce
- 1 cup scallions, chopped
- 4 tablespoons lemon juice
- 2 tablespoons apple cider vinegar
- 1/2 teaspoon cumin powder

Procedure:

1. First, boil the green beans in a large saucepan of salted water until they are just tender or about 2 minutes.
2. Then, drain and let the beans cool completely; then, transfer them to a salad bowl.
3. Now, toss the beans with the remaining ingredients.
4. Bon appétit!

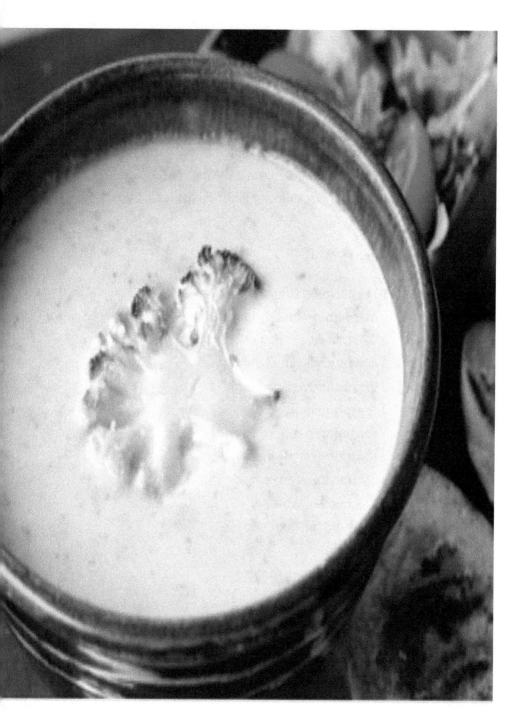

Servings: 4

Preparation Time: 10 minutes

Per Serving: Calories 202, Total Fat 8. 4g, Saturated Fat 4. 4g, Cholesterol 20mg, Sodium 1345mg, Total Carbohydrate 23. 2g, Dietary Fiber 7. 8g, Total Sugars 11. 3g, Protein 12. 6g

Ingredients:

- 10 cups vegetable broth or water
- 2 medium onions chopped
- 2 - 4 stalks leek thinly sliced
- 4 cloves garlic crushed
- 2 lbs cauliflower cut in big chunks
- 2 teaspoons salt
- 1 teaspoon pepper
- 2 teaspoons fresh basil
- 1/2 cup almond flour
- 1 1/3 cups of water
- 2 cups grated goat cheese
- 1 cup milk
- Salt and pepper to taste

Procedure:

1. First, add the first 8 ingredients (including basil) to the Instant Pot and lock lid.

2. Make sure the valve is set to Sealing and press Pressure Cooker (or Manual).
3. Then, set the time with the + /- button for 5 minutes.
4. While cooking, stir in flour and water until smooth.
5. When the IP beeps, flip the valve from Sealing to Venting, and when the pin drops, press Cancel and remove the lid.
6. Now, press the Sauté button and cook again, stirring frequently.
7. Whisk the flour-water mixture and add about half of it to the soup.
8. Use a hand blender to puree the soup. Or use a blender or food processor and put it back in the pan.
9. Press Cancel and add the cheese.
10. Then, stir until melted.
11. Do not cook after the cheese has gone in.
12. Now, add the milk, salt, and pepper to your taste.
13. Finally, serve with a pinch of grated cheese.

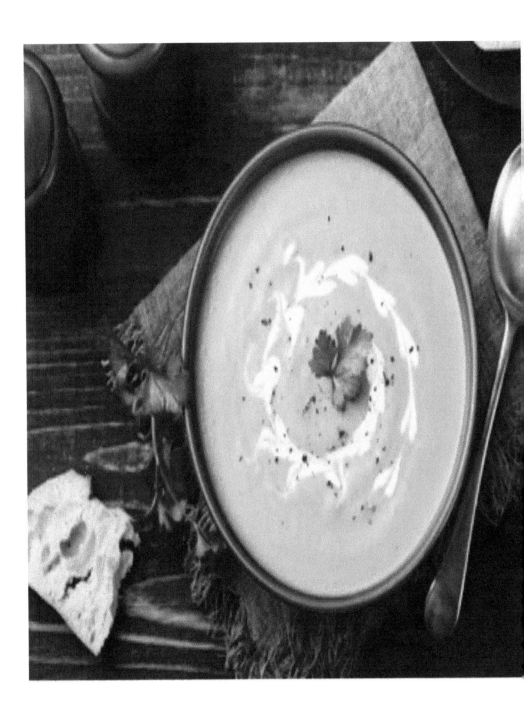

Servings: 4

Preparation Time: 10 minutes

Per Serving: Calories 415, Total Fat 41g, Saturated Fat 32. 9g, Cholesterol 31mg, Sodium 1064mg, Total Carbohydrate 11. 5g, Dietary Fiber 3. 3g, Total Sugars 5. 2g, Protein 5. 9g

Ingredients:

- 2 lbs pumpkins peeled and seeded 1/2-1inch cubes
- 2 teaspoons dried rosemary
- 2 cups vegetable broth or water
- 2 tablespoons almond flour
- 1/2 teaspoon grated cinnamon
- 1 teaspoon salt
- 2 cups of coconut milk
- 4 tablespoons butter

Procedure:

1. Start by mixing the pumpkin cubes, broth, rosemary, cinnamon, and salt in an Instant Pot. Lock the lid onto the pot.
2. Then, press Soup/Broth, Pressure Cooker, or Manual on High Pressure for 5 minutes with the Keep Warm setting off. The valve must be closed.
3. Use the Quick-release mode to return the pot pressure to normal.

4. Unlock the lid and open the pot. Add coconut milk.
5. Use an immersion blender to puree the soup right in the pot. Or work in halves to puree the soup in a covered blender. If necessary, pour all the soup back into the pan.
6. Now, press the Sauté button and set it for Low, 250°F. Set the timer for 5 minutes.
7. Bring the soup to a simmer, stirring often.
8. In the meantime, place the butter in a small bowl or measuring container and place it in the microwave in 5-second increments.
9. Use a fork to mix the flour and make a thin paste.
10. When the soup is boiling, whisk the butter mixture into the pan.
11. Then continue whisking until the soup is a bit thick, about 1 minute.
12. Finally, turn off the Sauté function and allow it to cool for a few minutes before serving.

Servings: 4

Preparation Time: 10 minutes

Per Serving: Calories 435, Total Fat 34. 3g, Saturated Fat 28g, Cholesterol 8mg, Sodium 1228mg, Total Carbohydrate 25. 1g, Dietary Fiber 7. 4g, Total Sugars 11. 2g, Protein 12. 2g

Ingredients:

- 3 cups chopped carrots
- 2 onions and sliced
- 1 tablespoon butter
- 1 cup chopped pumpkin
- 1/2 cup tomato, chopped
- Salt & pepper to taste
- 6 cups vegetable broth
- 2 teaspoons garlic powder
- 2 cups of coconut milk
- 2 tablespoons grated ginger
- 2 tablespoons turmeric powder

Procedure:

1. Set on Sauté mode and pour in the butter.
2. Now, add in the diced onion, carrots, and mix until combined.
3. Sauté for about 5 minutes or until the vegetables become soft.

4. Then, stir in the garlic powder, ginger turmeric powder, salt, and pepper.
5. After that, add in the pumpkin, tomatoes, broth, coconut milk, and stir to combine.
6. Lock the lid in place and close the steam vent.
7. Set on Manual or Pressure Cooker on High Pressure for 4 minutes.
8. Now, allow the Instant Pot to Natural-release for 5 minutes once the timer goes off.
9. Then, remove the lid and stir to combine.
10. Enjoy!

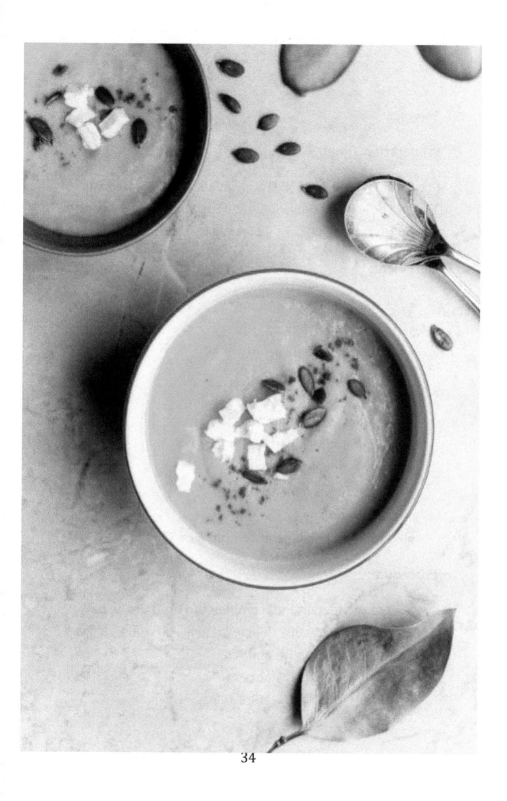

Tasty Coconut Tofu Soup

Servings: 4

Preparation Time: 10 minutes

Per Serving: Calories 238, Total Fat 19. 2g, Saturated Fat 13. 7g, Cholesterol 0mg, Sodium 31mg, Total Carbohydrate 10. 3g, Dietary Fiber 2. 9g, Total Sugars 5g, Protein 11g

Ingredients:

- 1 cup full fat coconut milk
- 2 tablespoons ginger
- 4 cups vegetable broth or water
- 1 pound tofu
- 4 whole red chills
- 1 tablespoon lemon zest
- Chopped fresh parsley for garnish
- Lime wedges for serving
- 2 teaspoons maple syrup
- 1 teaspoon salt
- 1/2 cup fresh lime juice from 2 or 3 limes

Procedure:

1. Set the Instant Pot, combine the broth, tofu, half the coconut milk, the ginger, chills (if using), lemon zest, maple syrup, and salt.
2. Lock lid on the Instant Pot.
3. Now, close the Pressure-release valve.

4. Select Manual or Pressure Cooker and set the pot at Low Pressure for 1 minute.
5. At the end of the cooking time, quickly release the pressure.
6. Then, stir in the remaining coconut milk and lime juice.
7. Now, divide the soup among two serving bowls.
8. Finally, garnish with parsley and serve with lime wedges alongside for squeezing.

Servings: 4

Preparation Time: 10 minutes

Per Serving: Calories 249, Total Fat 6. 8g, Saturated Fat 2. 7g, Cholesterol 8mg, Sodium 867mg, Total Carbohydrate 35. 8g, Dietary Fiber 5. 4g, Total Sugars 7. 2g, Protein 11. 3g

Ingredients:

- 2 cups fresh Swiss chard
- Pinch of salt & pepper
- 1 tablespoon butter
- 1 cup chopped parsnips
- 1 cup sliced leeks,
- 2 teaspoons garlic powder
- 1 tablespoon lemon zest
- 1/2 cup onion
- 1/2 cup millet
- 4 cups vegetable broth
- 1 cup of soy milk
- 1/4 cup lemon juice

Procedure:

1. First, heat the butter in an Instant Pot and select the Sauté function.

2. When butter melts, add the onion, parsnips, leeks, and garlic powder, and sauté until soft, about 5 minutes.
3. Now, add lemon zest, broth, and millet, salt, and pepper, and stir to combine.
4. Lock lid in place and turn the valve to Sealing.
5. Then, press the Pressure Cooker button and set the cooking time for 20 minutes at High Pressure.
6. When the Instant Pot beeps, let it go for 10 minutes.
7. Now, release the remaining pressure naturally and open the pot when the pin drops.
8. Once the millet is cooked and soft, stir in the soy milk, lemon juice, and Swiss chard.
9. Now, stir until the Swiss chard is wilted.
10. Lock lid and press hit pressure (or Manual). Set the cooking time to 4 minutes.
11. When it's done, take a quick release (pin drop), open the Instant Pot.
12. Finally, serve immediately and enjoy! Soup can be frozen and reheated as desired

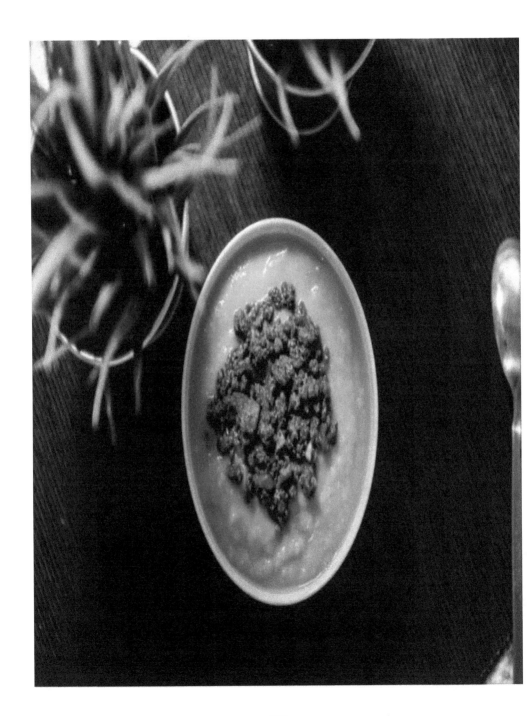

Amazing Turmeric Bean Soup

Servings: 12

Preparation Time: 50 minutes

Ingredients:

- 4 carrots, chopped
- 6 tbsps olive oil
- 2 sweet potatoes, chopped
- 4 garlic cloves, minced
- 8 tomatoes, chopped
- 2 (31-oz) cans white beans, drained
- 12 cups vegetable broth
- 2 bay leafs
- 1/2 tsp turmeric
- 2 tsps ground cayenne pepper
- 2/3 cup whole-wheat pasta
- 2 yellow bell peppers, chopped
- 1 onion, chopped
- Salt to taste

Procedure:

1. First, heat the oil in a pot over medium heat. Place onion, carrots, sweet potato, bell pepper, and garlic.
2. Now, cook for 5 minutes.
3. Then, add in tomatoes, broth, bay leaf, salt, and cayenne pepper.

4. Stir and bring to a boil.
5. Lower the heat and simmer for 10 minutes.
6. Put in white beans and simmer for 15 more minutes.
7. Now, cook the pasta in a pot with boiling salted water and turmeric for 8-10 minutes, until pasta is al dente.
8. Then strain and transfer to the soup.
9. Discard the bay leaf. Spoon into a bowl and serve.

VEGETABLE & SIDE DISHES

Servings: 8

Preparation Time: 15 minutes

Ingredients:

- 2 lbs extra-firm tofu, crumbled
- 6 green onions, minced
- 1/2 cup shelled sunflower seeds
- 2 celery stalks, chopped
- 2 medium carrots, chopped
- 8 lettuce leaves
- 8 slices ripe tomato
- 1 cup tofu mayonnaise
- 16 slices whole-grain bread

Procedure:

1. First, place the tofu in a bowl. Stir in carrot, celery, green onions, and sunflower seeds.
2. Then, mix in mayonnaise, salt, and pepper.
3. Toast the bread slices.
4. Now, spread the tofu mixture onto 4 bread slices.
5. Layer a tomato slice and lettuce leaf. Top each sandwich with a bread slice and cut diagonally.
6. Finally, serve immediately.

Servings: 8

Preparation Time: 40 minutes

Ingredients:

- 8 tbsps plant butter, melted
- 8 garlic cloves, minced
- 3 lbs baby potatoes
- 4 tbsps grated plant-based Parmesan
- 6 tbsps chopped chives
- Salt and black pepper to taste

Procedure:

1. Preheat the oven to 400 F.
2. Take a bowl, mix butter, garlic, chives, salt, pepper, and plant Parmesan cheese.
3. Now, toss the potatoes in the butter mixture until coated.
4. Spread the mixture into a baking sheet, cover with foil, and roast for 30 minutes.
5. Then, remove the potatoes from the oven and toss in the remaining butter mixture.
6. Finally, serve.

Servings: 8

Preparation Time: 25 minutes

Ingredients:

- 2 cups grated plant-based Parmesan
- 2 cups cashew cream cheese
- 2 oz. tofu, chopped into small bits
- 2 cups red and yellow bell peppers
- 2 tbsps chili paste, mild
- 4 tbsps melted plant butter

Procedure:

1. First, preheat the oven to 400 F. Use a knife to cut the bell peppers into two (lengthwise) and remove the core.
2. Take a bowl, mix tofu, cashew cream cheese, chili paste, and melted butter until smooth.
3. Spoon the cheese mixture into the bell peppers and use the back of the spoon to level the filling in the peppers.
4. Now, grease a baking sheet with cooking spray and arrange the stuffed peppers on the sheet.
5. Then, sprinkle the plant-based Parmesan cheese on top and bake the peppers for 15-20 minutes until the peppers are golden brown and the cheese melted.
6. Lastly, remove onto a serving platter and serve warm.

Easy Three-Lentil Curry

Servings: 4

Preparation Time: 10 minutes

Per Serving: Calories 340, Total Fat 21. 1g, Saturated Fat 16. 3g, Cholesterol 0mg, Sodium 390mg, Total Carbohydrate 30. 8g, Dietary Fiber 10. 8g, Total Sugars 5. 7g, Protein 10. 4g

Ingredients:

- 8 cups of water
- 2 bay leaves
- 2 teaspoons ginger powder
- 1 tablespoon garam masala
- 2 teaspoons cumin powder
- 1/2 teaspoon turmeric powder
- 1/2 teaspoon table salt
- 1 tablespoon coconut oil
- 1/2 teaspoon paprika
- 1 cup coconut cream
- 2 cinnamon stick 4-inch stick
- 4 green cardamom pods
- 2 teaspoons garlic powder
- 1 cup red tomatoes chopped
- 1/2 cup red lentils
- 1/2 cup brown lentils
- 1/2 cup green lentils
- 1/2 cup

Procedure:

1. Press Sauté, set the time for 5 minutes.
2. Now, add coconut oil to the Instant Pot.
3. Add the garlic powder, ginger powder, garam masala, cumin powder, turmeric powder, salt, paprika, cinnamon stick, cardamom pods, and bay leaves.
4. Then, stir until fragrant, about 1 minute. Add the tomatoes and cook, often stirring until it just begins to break down, 1 to 2 minutes.
5. Turn off the Sauté function.
6. Now, stir in the red lentils, brown lentils, and green lentils until coated in the spices.
7. After, stir in the water and lock the lid onto the Instant Pot.
8. Press Pressure Cook on Max Pressure for 16 minutes with the Keep Warm setting off.
9. Use the Quick-release method to bring the Instant Pot pressure back to normal.
10. Now, unlatch the lid and open the Instant Pot.
11. Then, remove and discard the cinnamon stick, cardamom pods, and bay leaves.
12. Now, stir in the cream until uniform, then set the lid askew over the Instant Pot for 5 minutes to blend the flavors.
13. Lastly, stir again before serving.

Servings: 4

Preparation Time: 5 minutes

Per Serving: Calories 268, Total Fat 2. 7g, Saturated Fat 0. 3g, Cholesterol 0mg, Sodium 555mg, Total Carbohydrate 50. 6g, Dietary Fiber 13g, Total Sugars 11. 8g, Protein 14g

Ingredients:

- 1 cup kidney beans rinsed and drained
- 1 cup chickpea beans rinsed and drained
- 2 teaspoons paprika
- 1 tablespoon ground mustard
- 1 cup pinto beans rinsed and drained
- 2 cups of water
- 1 cup tomato paste
- 2 teaspoons honey

Procedure:

1. First, add the kidney beans, pinto beans, chickpeas beans, water, tomato paste, honey, ground mustard, and paprika.
2. Now, lock the lid into place and turn the valve to "Sealing. " Select Manual or Pressure Cook and adjust the pressure to High.
3. Then, set the time for 8 minutes.

4. When cooking ends, let the pressure release naturally for 15 minutes, then turn the valve to "Venting" to quickly release the remaining pressure.
5. Unlock and remove the lid and stir well before serving.

Servings: 4

Preparation Time: 10 minutes

Per Serving: Calories 269, Total Fat 1. 6g, Saturated Fat 0. 3g, Cholesterol 0mg, Sodium 255mg, Total Carbohydrate 55. 2g, Dietary Fiber 7. 4g, Total Sugars 1. 6g, Protein 9. 9g

Ingredients:

- 1 cup chopped onions
- 1 cup brown lentils
- 1 cup of brown rice
- 2 cups of water
- 1 cup low sodium vegetable broth
- 1 tablespoon rosemary
- 2 teaspoons garlic powder
- 1 cup navy beans pre-soaked or quick-soaked

Procedure:

1. In your Instant Pot, sauté the onions in the vegetable broth and garlic powder.
2. First, heat the broth on medium and statue the onion for about 4 minutes until translucent, then add the garlic powder for another 30 seconds.
3. Now, add the rest of the ingredients to Instant Pot, and stir it well.

4. Then, close the lid, and seal the vent Instant Pot.
5. Set the cooker for 23 minutes, and cook at High pressure on the Manual setting.
6. Release the pressure naturally.
7. Finally, serve and season as desired.

Servings: 4

Preparation Time: 15 minutes

Per Serving: Calories 186, Total Fat 3. 5g, Saturated Fat 0. 5g, Cholesterol 0mg, Sodium 602mg, Total Carbohydrate 29. 9g, Dietary Fiber 11. 6g, Total Sugars 5. 5g, Protein 11. 4g

Ingredients:

- 1 teaspoon ground red pepper
- 1 tablespoon ground cumin
- 2 tomatoes, chopped
- 2 tablespoons tomato paste
- 2 small onions, chopped
- 2 cups of water
- 1 cup fava beans, drained
- 2 tablespoons finely chopped parsley
- 2 teaspoons olive oil
- 1 teaspoon salt
- 3 teaspoons ground black pepper

Procedure:

1. Take your Instant Pot, sauté olive oil and add onions.
2. Cook and stir for 2 minutes.
3. Now, add chopped tomatoes and tomato paste; cook until tomatoes are mushy, about 4 minutes.

4. Then, pour fava beans into Instant Pot. Add 1 cup water, cumin, salt, black pepper, and ground red pepper; stir well.
5. After that, close the lid, and seal the vent Instant Pot. Set the cooker for 23 minutes, and cook at High pressure on the Manual setting.
6. Now, release the pressure naturally.
7. Lastly, stir in parsley.

Servings: 4

Preparation Time: 15 minutes

Per Serving: Calories 240, Total Fat 4. 8g, Saturated Fat 1g, Cholesterol 0mg, Sodium 325mg, Total Carbohydrate 38. 8g, Dietary Fiber 4. 5g, Total Sugars 5. 8g, Protein 13. 4g

Ingredients:

- 1 cup split pigeon pea
- 1 tablespoon vegetable oil
- 1/2 teaspoon cumin seeds
- 2 green chili peppers sliced (optional
- 1/2 teaspoon red chili powder
- 1/2 teaspoon ginger powder
- 1 teaspoon garlic powder
- 1/4 teaspoon turmeric powder
- 2 tomatoes large, chopped
- 4 cups of water
- 1/2 teaspoon garam masala
- 2 cups spinach chopped
- 1/2 teaspoon salt

Procedure:

1. Start the Instant Pot in Sauté mode and heat vegetable oil in it.
2. Now, add cumin seeds, green chili, ginger powder, and garlic powder.

3. Sauté for 30 seconds until garlic turns golden brown, then add chopped tomatoes and spices.
4. Then add the split pigeon pea and water.
5. Stir well.
6. Press Cancel and close the Instant Pot lid with the vent in the Sealing position.
7. Now, press Manual or Pressure Cook mode for 3 minutes.
8. When the Instant Pot beeps, do a Quick Pressure Release.
9. After, that open the lid and add chopped spinach and garam masala.
10. Press Sauté mode. Simmer for 2 minutes until the dal starts boiling, and spinach is mixed with the lentils.
11. Finally, spinach split pigeon pea is ready to be served.

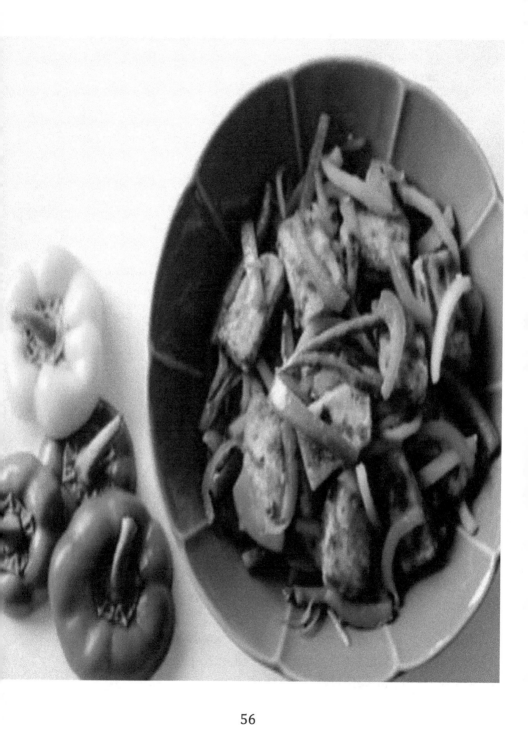

Servings: 4

Preparation Time: 15 minutes

Per Serving: Calories: 154; Fat: 13.7g; Carbs: 2.9g; Protein: 0.5g

Ingredients:

- 4 cloves garlic, minced
- 6 tablespoons olive oil
- Salt and freshly ground black pepper, to taste
- 8 bell peppers, seeded and slice into strips
- 4 tablespoons fresh cilantro, roughly chopped
- 2 teaspoons cayenne pepper
- 8 tablespoons dry white wine

Procedure:

1. Take a saucepan, heat the oil over medium-high heat.
2. Once hot, sauté the peppers for about 4 minutes or until tender and fragrant.
3. Then, sauté the garlic for about 1 minute until aromatic.
4. Now, add in the salt, black pepper, and cayenne pepper; continue to sauté, adding the wine, for about 6 minutes more until tender and cooked through.
5. Then, taste and adjust the seasonings.
6. Finally, top with fresh cilantro and serve. Bon appétit!

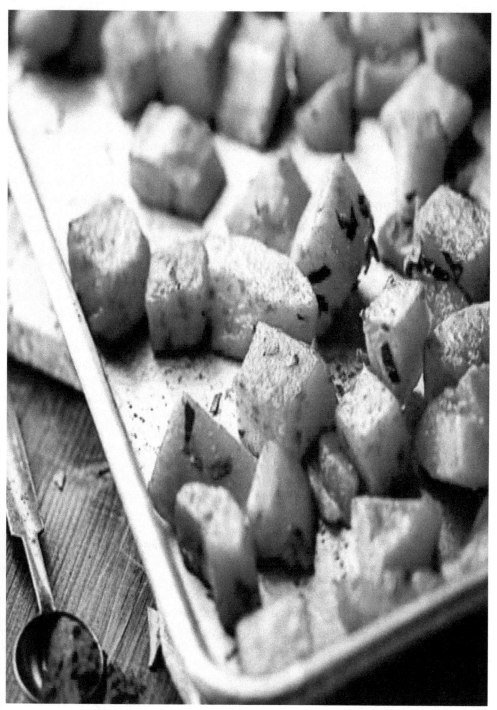

Servings: 8

Preparation Time: 25 minutes

Per Serving: Calories: 247; Fat: 16.5g; Carbs: 23.8g; Protein: 4.3g

Ingredients:

- 1 teaspoon ground allspice
- 3 pounds butternut squash, peeled, seeded, and diced
- 1/2 cup dry white wine
- Sea salt and ground black pepper, to taste
- 2 teaspoons paprika
- 4 tablespoons dark soy sauce
- 1 teaspoon ground cumin
- 8 tablespoons olive oil
- 2 teaspoons mustard seeds

Procedure:

1. Start by preheating your oven to 420 degrees F.
2. Then, toss the squash with the remaining ingredients.
3. Now, roast the butternut squash for about 25 minutes or until tender and caramelized.
4. Finally, serve warm and enjoy!

Servings: 8

Preparation Time: 10 minutes

Per Serving: Calories: 217; Fat: 13g; Carbs: 20.3g; Protein: 8.7g

Ingredients:

- 4 pounds cauliflower florets
- Sea salt and ground black pepper, to taste
- 6 tablespoons soy sauce
- 4 cloves garlic, minced
- 2 cups water
- 4 tablespoons lemon juice
- 10 tablespoons tahini

Procedure:

1. Take a large saucepan, bring the water to a boil; then, add in the cauliflower and cook for about 6 minutes or until fork-tender; drain, season with salt and pepper, and reserve.
2. Then, in a mixing bowl, thoroughly combine the soy sauce, tahini, garlic, and lemon juice.
3. Now, spoon the sauce over the cauliflower florets and serve.
4. Bon appétit!

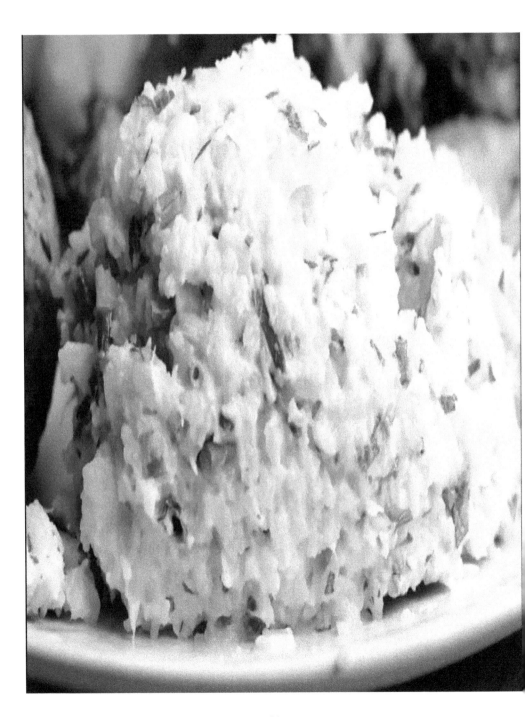

61

Amazing Herb Cauliflower Mash

Servings: 8

Preparation Time: 25 minutes

Per Serving: Calories: 167; Fat: 13g; Carbs: 11.3g; Protein: 4.4g

Ingredients:

- 3 pounds cauliflower florets
- 8 cloves garlic, sliced
- 4 tablespoons fresh parsley, roughly chopped
- 1/2 cup plain oat milk, unsweetened
- 8 tablespoons vegan butter
- Sea salt and ground black pepper, to taste

Procedure:

1. First, steam the cauliflower florets for about 20 minutes; set it aside to cool.
2. Take a saucepan, melt the vegan butter over moderately high heat; now, sauté the garlic for about 1 minute or until aromatic.
3. Now, add the cauliflower florets to your food processor, followed by the sautéed garlic, salt, black pepper, and oat milk.
4. Then, puree until everything is well incorporated.
5. Finally, garnish with fresh parsley leaves and serve hot. Bon appétit!

MAIN DISHES

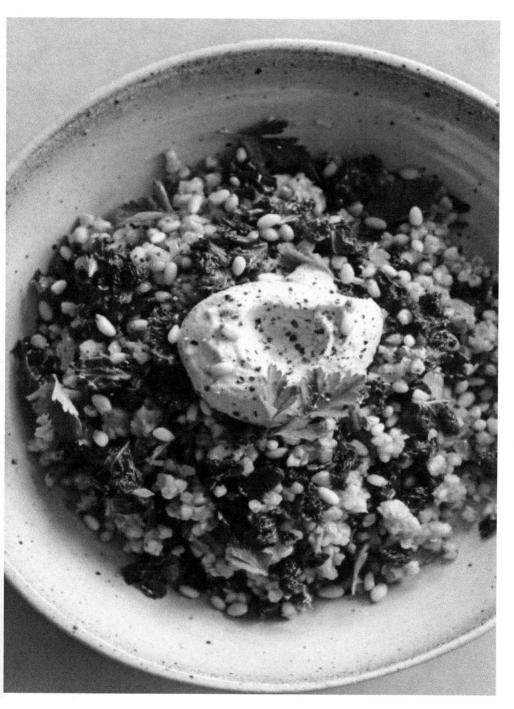

Servings: 8

Preparation Time: 25 minutes

Ingredients:

- 4 cups vegetable stock
- 2/3 cup chopped fresh parsley
- 2 cups buckwheat groats
- 1/2 cup pine nuts
- 4 tbsps olive oil
- 1 onion, chopped

Procedure:

1. First, put the groats and vegetable stock in a pot.
2. Bring to a boil, then lower the heat and simmer for 15 minutes.
3. Now, heat a skillet over medium heat. Place in the pine nuts and toast for 2-3 minutes, shaking often.
4. Heat the oil in the same skillet and sauté the onion for 3 minutes until translucent.
5. Once the groats are ready, fluff them using a fork.
6. Then, mix in pine nuts, onion, and parsley.
7. After sprinkle with salt and pepper.
8. Lastly, serve.

Servings: 8

Preparation Time: 25 minutes

Ingredients:

- 4 celery stalks, sliced
- 2 cups button mushrooms, sliced
- Chopped fresh parsley
- Sea salt to taste
- 6 garlic cloves, minced
- 1 cup vegetable broth
- 1 cup raisins
- 1/2 cup plant butter
- 2 onions, chopped
- 2 cups chopped walnuts
- 4 cups cooked quinoa
- 2 tsps Italian seasoning

Procedure:

1. Set a skillet over medium heat, melt the butter.
2. Sauté the onion, garlic, celery, and mushrooms for 5 minutes until tender, stirring occasionally.
3. Now, pour in broth, raisins, and walnuts.
4. Bring to a boil, then lower the heat and simmer for 5 minutes.
5. Then, stir in quinoa, Italian seasoning, and salt.
6. Now, cook for another 4 minutes.
7. Finally, serve garnished with parsley.

Servings: 12

Preparation Time: 30 minutes

Ingredients:

- 6 tbsps coconut oil
- 2 tsps ground ginger
- 4 tbsps curry powder
- 2 onions, chopped
- 6 cups water
- 4 garlic cloves, sliced
- Salt and black pepper to taste
- 2 cups dried green lentils

Procedure:

1. Set your IP to Sauté.
2. Now, add coconut oil, curry powder, ginger, onion, and garlic.
3. Cook for 3 minutes.
4. Then, stir in green lentils.
5. Pour in water. Lock the lid and set the time to 10 minutes on High.
6. Once ready, perform a natural pressure release for 10 minutes.
7. Unlock the lid and season with salt and pepper.
8. Now, serve.

Tasty Tomato Sauce with Pumpkin

Servings: 4

Preparation Time: 10 minutes

Per Serving: Calories191, Total Fat 7. 6g, Saturated Fat 1. 7g, Cholesterol 0mg, Sodium 840mg, Total Carbohydrate 28. 9g, Dietary Fiber 11. 4g, Total Sugars, Protein 6g

Ingredients:

- 1 tablespoon dried basil
- 1 teaspoon salt and pepper
- 2 teaspoons garlic minced
- 1 cup avocado oil
- 2 cups pumpkin
- 2 small onions diced
- 1/4 cup fresh coriander washed and chopped
- 2 cups crushed tomatoes
- 2 tablespoons tomato paste

Procedure:

1. Set the Instant Pot to Sauté.
2. Now, add avocado oil and wait one minute to heat up.
3. Add the onion and garlic, sauté for one minute.
4. Stir often.
5. Then, add the pumpkin, coriander, and sauté for one minute.
6. Stir often.

7. After then, add the crushed tomatoes, tomato paste, dried basil, salt, and pepper.
8. Now, stir well.
9. Cover the Instant Pot and lock it in.
10. Then, set the Manual or Pressure Cook timer for 10 minutes.
11. Make sure the timer is set to "Sealing."
12. Once the timer reaches zero, quickly release the pressure.
13. Enjoy!

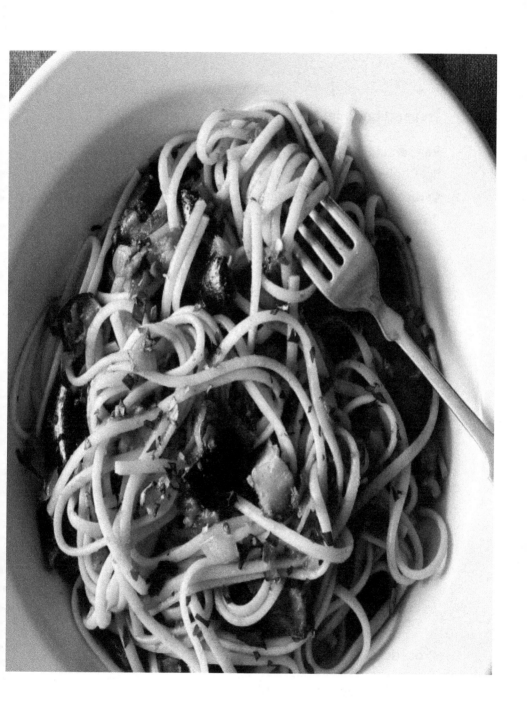

Servings: 4

Preparation Time: 5 minutes

Per Serving: Calories 405, Total Fat 14. 2g, Saturated Fat 9. 8g, Cholesterol 62mg, Sodium 1443mg, Total Carbohydrate 56. 1g, Dietary Fiber 5. 2g, Total Sugars 8g, Protein 16. 1g

Ingredients:

- 2 medium zucchinis, chopped
- 4 cloves of garlic minced
- 2 cups juice
- 2 tablespoons tomato paste
- 1 cup vegetable broth
- 2 teaspoons dried thyme
- 2 tablespoons coconut oil
- 2 teaspoons dried oregano
- 2 teaspoons kosher salt
- 2 onions finely diced
- Shredded goat cheese for garnish
- 1/2 teaspoon pepper
- 1 cup diced tomatoes
- 2 cups eggplant, diced
- 2 tablespoons corn-starch

Procedure:

1. First, add coconut oil to the Instant Pot.

2. Using the display panel select the Sauté function.
3. When oil gets hot, add onion to the Instant Pot and sauté for 3 minutes.
4. Now, add zucchini and cook for 3 minutes more.
5. Add garlic and tomato paste and cook for 1-2 minutes more.
6. Then, add vegetable broth and seasonings to the Instant pot and deglaze by using a wooden spoon to scrape the brown bits from the bottom of the pot.
7. Add tomatoes to the Instant Pot and stir.
8. Now, add eggplant to the Instant Pot, turning once to coat.
9. Turn the Instant pot off by selecting Cancel, and then secure the lid, making sure the vent is closed.
10. Using the display panel, select the Manual or Pressure Cook function.
11. After, use the + /- keys and program the Instant Pot for 20 minutes.
12. When the time is up, let the pressure naturally release for 15 minutes, then quickly release the remaining pressure.
13. Take a small bowl, mix 1/4 cup of Instant pot juices and corn-starch.
14. Stir into the pot until thickened.
15. Finally, serve hot topped with shredded cheese.

Servings: 4

Preparation Time: 5 minutes

Per Serving: Calories 383, Total Fat 4. 2g, Saturated Fat 0. 9g, Cholesterol 1mg, Sodium 1269mg, Total Carbohydrate 73. 8g, Dietary Fiber 5g, Total Sugars 9g, Protein 12. 4g

Ingredients:

- 4 cups of water
- 4 cups dried rigatoni
- 2 teaspoons garlic powder
- 2 teaspoons grated lemon zest
- 1 cup broccoli
- 1/4 teaspoon crushed red pepper flakes
- 1 cup pasta sauce
- 1 cup pitted Kalamata olives sliced
- 1 teaspoon fine sea salt
- 1/2 teaspoon ground black pepper

Procedure:

1. First, combine all of the ingredients in the inner cooking pot and stir to coat the pasta.
2. Lock the lid into place and turn the valve to "Sealing. "

3. Now, select Manual or Pressure Cook and adjust the pressure to High. Set the time for 5 minutes.
4. When cooking ends, carefully turn the valve to "Venting" to quickly release the pressure.
5. Unlock and remove the lid.
6. Then, serve hot.

Servings: 4

Preparation Time: 5 minutes

Per Serving: Calories 499, Total Fat 31g, Saturated Fat 25. 8g, Cholesterol 23mg, Sodium 337mg, Total Carbohydrate 49. 2g, Dietary Fiber 10g, Total Sugars 12. 4g, Protein 12. 8g

Ingredients:

- 2 cups of coconut milk
- 2 bell peppers seeded and cut into chunks
- 2 cups basil
- 2 leeks green part only, cut into chunks
- 1 cup broccoli florets
- 2 cups green peas
- 2 cups noodles
- 2 teaspoons garlic powder
- 1/2 teaspoon salt
- 1 cup of water

Procedure:

1. Take a blender, add coconut milk, basil, bell pepper, leek, garlic powder, and salt.
2. Blend until smooth.
3. Now, pour the sauce into the inner pot and add the water.

4. Select Sauté and adjust to High heat. Bring just to a simmer, then turn the Instant Pot off.
5. Break up the noodles into 3 or 4 pieces and place them in the pot in a single layer as much as possible.
6. After then, layer the broccoli over the noodles.
7. Lock the lid into place.
8. Now, select Pressure Cook or Manual, and adjust the pressure to Low and the time to 25 minutes.
9. After cooking, quickly release the pressure.
10. Unlock the lid.
11. Gently stir the mixture until the broccoli and peas are coated with sauce.
12. Lastly, ladle into bowls and serve immediately.

Servings: 4

Preparation Time: 5 minutes

Per Serving: Calories 115, Total Fat 4. 1g, Saturated Fat 2. 2g, Cholesterol 10mg, Sodium 893mg, Total Carbohydrate 13. 9, Dietary Fiber 3. 6g 13%, Total Sugars 6. 1g, Protein 8. 5g

Ingredients:

- 1/4 cup finely chopped onion
- 1/2 cup crushed tomatoes
- 2 teaspoons Italian seasoning blend
- 2 teaspoons garlic powder
- 2 tablespoons fresh parsley
- 1 teaspoon dried basil
- 2 tablespoons grated Parmesan cheese
- 1 teaspoon of sea salt
- 1 teaspoon ground black pepper
- 1/2 cup vegetable broth
- 2 cloves garlic minced
- 2 cups mushrooms
- ½1 tablespoon avocado oil
- 2 bay leafs
- 2 cups spaghetti squash washed and dried
- 2 tablespoons tomato paste

Procedure:

1. First, select Sauté (Normal); once the pot is hot, add the avocado oil, mushrooms, garlic, and onions.
2. Sauté, stirring continuously, for about 5 minutes or until the mushrooms are browned.
3. Now, add the crushed tomatoes, Italian seasoning, garlic powder, basil, sea salt, black pepper, and vegetable broth to the pot.
4. Using a wooden spoon, stir and scrape the bottom of the pot to loosen any browned bits. Add the bay leaf.
5. Using a paring knife, pierce the spaghetti squash 4 or 5 times on each side to create holes for venting the steam.
6. Then, place the squash in the pot and on top of the sauce.
7. Cover, lock the lid, and flip the steam release handle to the sealing position.
8. After, select Manual or Pressure Cook (High) and set the cooking time to 8 minutes.
9. When the cooking time is complete, allow the pressure to release naturally for 20 minutes and then quickly release the remaining pressure.
10. Then, open the lid.
11. Using a slotted spoon, carefully transfer the squash to a cutting board and set it aside to cool.
12. Now, add the tomato paste to the pot and stir.

13. Select Sauté (Less or Low), replace the lid, and let the sauce simmer for 6 minutes.
14. While the sauce is simmering, slice the cooled squash in half and use a spoon to scoop out the seeds.
15. Using a fork, scrape the flesh to create the noodles.
16. After, that transfer the noodles to a colander to drain, pressing down on the noodles with paper towels to expel any excess moisture.
17. Transfer the noodles to a serving platter.
18. Now, remove and discard the bay leaf.
19. Then, ladle the sauce over top of the noodles and garnish with Parmesan and parsley.
20. Lastly, serve warm.

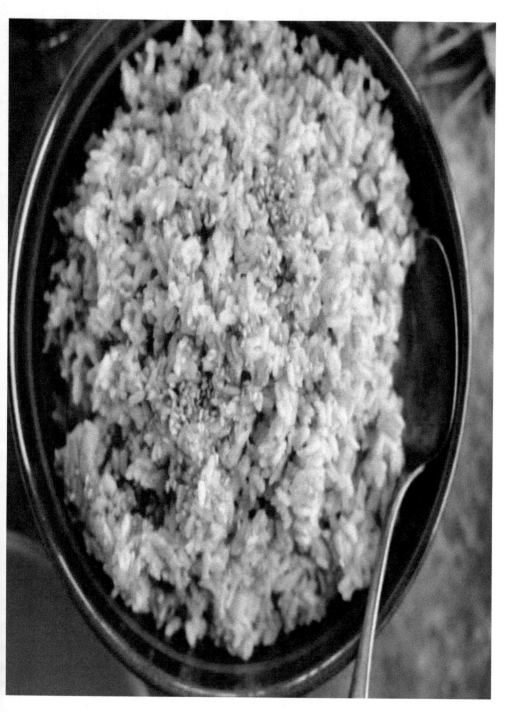

Servings: 8

Preparation Time: 30 minutes

Per Serving: Calories: 318; Fat: 8.8g; Carbs: 53.4g; Protein: 5.6g

Ingredients:

- 3 cups brown rice, rinsed
- 4 tablespoons olive oil
- 2 teaspoons garlic, minced
- Sea salt and ground black pepper, to taste
- 2 (2-inch) pieces of ginger, peeled and minced
- 1 teaspoon cumin seeds

Procedure:

1. First, place the brown rice in a saucepan and cover it with cold water by 2 inches.
2. Bring to a boil.
3. Turn the heat to a simmer and continue to cook for about 30 minutes or until tender.
4. Take a sauté pan, heat the olive oil over medium-high heat.
5. Once hot, cook the garlic, ginger, and cumin seeds until aromatic.
6. Now, stir the garlic/ginger mixture into the hot rice; season with salt and pepper, and serve immediately. Bon appétit!

Servings: 8

Preparation Time: 20 minutes

Per Serving: Calories: 380; Fat: 11.1g; Carbs: 59g; Protein: 14.4g

Ingredients:

- A pinch of grated nutmeg
- 12 prunes, chopped
- 2 cups almond milk
- 4 cups water
- A pinch of ground cloves
- 12 dates, pitted and chopped
- A pinch of sea salt
- 8 tablespoons almonds, slivered
- 3 cups steel-cut oats, soaked overnight

Procedure:

1. Take a deep saucepan, bring the steel cut oats, almond milk, and water to a boil.
2. Now, add in the nutmeg, cloves, and salt.
3. Immediately turn the heat to a simmer, cover, and continue to cook for about 15 minutes or until they've softened.
4. Then, spoon the grits into four serving bowls; top them with the almonds, dates, and prunes.
5. Bon appétit!

Servings: 16

Preparation Time: 10 minutes

Per Serving: Calories: 174; Fat: 9.1g; Carbs: 18.5g; Protein: 6.4g

Ingredients:

- 1 teaspoon ground cumin
- 1/2 teaspoon ground bay laurel
- 1 teaspoon red pepper flakes
- Sea salt and ground black pepper, to taste
- 4 tablespoons extra-virgin olive oil
- 2 teaspoons dried onion powder
- 4 tablespoons lemon juice
- 32 ounces chickpeas, boiled and drained
- 2 teaspoons parsley flakes
- 4 cloves of garlic, crushed
- 1/2 cup good-quality tahini

Procedure:

1. First, blitz all the ingredients in your blender or food processor until your desired consistency is reached.
2. Now, place in your refrigerator until ready to serve.
3. Then, serve with toasted pita wedges or chips. Bon appétit!

Traditional Asian Green Peas Stir-Fry

Servings: 8

Preparation Time: 10 minutes

Per Serving: Calories: 184; Fat: 8.7g; Carbs: 20.2g; Protein: 7.1g

Ingredients:

- 4 tablespoons scallions
- 1 teaspoon dried dill
- 2 pounds green peas, fresh or thawed
- 4 tablespoons pine nuts, chopped
- 4 tablespoons soy sauce
- 4 tablespoons peanut oil
- 8 garlic cloves, pressed
- 1/2 teaspoon red pepper, flakes
- 1 teaspoon Five-spice powder

Procedure:

1. First, heat the peanut oil in a wok until sizzling.
2. Now, stir-fry the garlic and scallions for 2 minutes or until crisp-tender.
3. Then, add in the dried dill and continue to cook for 30 seconds more or until fragrant.
4. After, add in the green peas and stir-fry over high heat for about 3 minutes until lightly charred.
5. Then, stir in the red pepper, Five-spice powder, and soy sauce; stir-fry for 1 minute more.
6. Lastly, garnish with chopped pine nuts and enjoy.

Servings: 8

Preparation Time: 10 minutes

Per Serving: Calories: 344; Fat: 22.7g; Carbs: 24.5g; Protein: 14.2g

Ingredients:

- 32 ounces sweet peas
- 8 tablespoons shallots, chopped
- 2 Persian cucumbers, diced
- 8 tablespoons extra-virgin olive oil
- 2 tablespoons fresh lemon juice
- 2 teaspoons Dijon mustard
- 2 teaspoons garlic, minced
- 2 teaspoons fresh dill, chopped
- 4 tablespoons fresh parsley, chopped
- 12 ounces tofu, pressed and cubed

Procedure:

1. First, cook the green peas in a pot of lightly salted water for 5 to 6 minutes.
2. Let it cool completely.

3. Now, add the peas to a salad bowl; add in the shallot, cucumber, olive oil, lemon juice, mustard, garlic, dill, and parsley.
4. Gently toss to combine and top with the cubed tofu.
5. Lastly, serve at room temperature or place in your refrigerator until ready to serve.

DESSERTS

Delicious Mango Muffins with Chocolate Chips

Servings: 24

Preparation Time: 40 minutes

Ingredients:

- 4 tbsps almond butter
- 2 tsps apple cider vinegar
- 2 tsps pure vanilla extract
- 2 1/2 cups whole-wheat flour
- 1 cup rolled oats
- 4 medium mangoes, chopped
- 1/2 cup coconut sugar
- 2 cups non-dairy milk
- A pinch of salt
- 1/2 cup dark chocolate chips
- 2 tsps baking powder
- 1 tsp baking soda
- 1 cup unsweetened cocoa powder
- 1/2 cup sesame seeds

Procedure:

1. Preheat oven to 360 F.
2. Take a food processor, put the mangoes, milk, almond butter, vinegar, and vanilla.
3. Blend until smooth.

4. Take a bowl, combine the flour, oats, sugar, baking powder, baking soda, cocoa powder, sesame seeds, salt, and chocolate chips.
5. Now, pour into the mango mixture and mix.
6. Scoop into greased muffin cups and bake for 20-25 minutes.
7. Then, let it cool completely before removing it from the cups.

Servings: 6

Preparation Time: 15 minutes

Ingredients:

- 1 cup pure date sugar
- 1 1/2 cups of plant butter, softened
- 2 tsps pure vanilla extract
- 1 1/2 cups of poppy seeds, lightly toasted
- 4 tbsps pure maple syrup
- 4 cups whole-grain flour

Procedure:

1. First, beat the butter and sugar in a bowl until creamy and fluffy.
2. Now, add in vanilla, and maple syrup, blend. Stir in flour and poppy seeds.
3. Wrap the dough in a cylinder and cover it with plastic foil.
4. Then, let chill in the fridge.
5. Preheat oven to 330 F.
6. Now, cut the dough into thin circles and arrange it on a baking sheet.
7. Bake for 12 minutes until light brown.
8. Lastly, let it completely cool before serving.

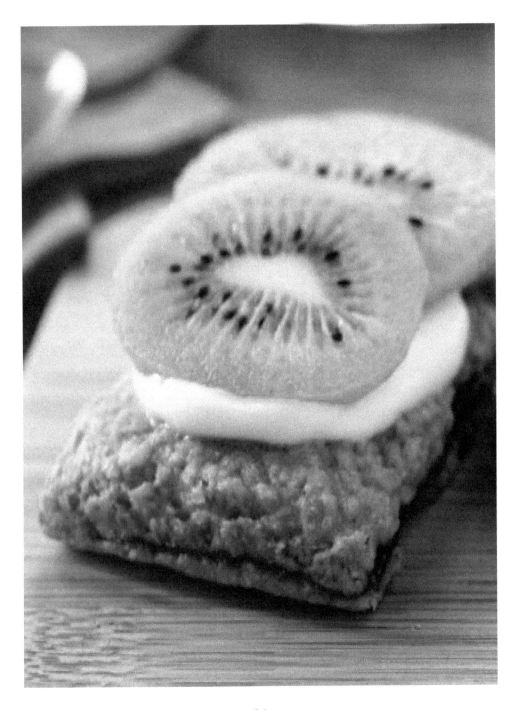

Servings: 18

Preparation Time: 5 minutes

Ingredients:

- 1 tsp vanilla extract
- 1/2 cup chopped peanuts
- 2 tbsps maple syrup
- 4 kiwis, mashed
- 4 cups old-fashioned rolled oats
- 1 tsp salt

Procedure:

1. Preheat oven to 360 F.
2. Take a bowl, add kiwi, maple syrup, and vanilla, and stir.
3. Now, mix in oats, salt, and peanuts.
4. Then, pour into a greased baking dish and bake for 25-30 minutes until crisp.
5. In the end, let it completely cool and slice into bars to serve.

Servings: 8

Preparation Time: 20 minutes + cooling time

Ingredients:

- 5 tbsps pure date sugar
- 12 oz. cashew cream cheese
- 2 ripe mangoes, chopped
- 1 1/3 cups toasted rolled oats
- 6 tsps agar agar powder
- 1/2 cup plant butter, melted
- 1/2 cup coconut milk
- 2 lemons, zested and juiced
- 1/2 cup just-boiled water

Procedure:

1. First, process the oats, butter, and date sugar in a blender until smooth.
2. Now, pour the mixture into a greased 9-inch springform pan and press the mixture onto the bottom of the pan.
3. Refrigerate for 30 minutes until firm while you make the filling.
4. Take a large bowl, using an electric mixer, whisk the cashew cream cheese until smooth.
5. Beat in coconut milk, lemon zest, and lemon juice.

6. Now, mix the boiled water and agar-agar powder until dissolved and whisk this mixture into the creamy mix. Fold in the mango.
7. Then, remove the cake pan from the fridge and pour in the mango mixture.
8. Shake the pan to ensure smooth layering on top.
9. Refrigerate further for at least 3 hours.
10. Finally, remove the cheesecake from the fridge, release the cake pan, slice, and serve.

Servings: 8

Preparation Time: 15-30 minutes

Per Serving: Calories 466 Fats 29. 9g Carbs 47. 8g Protein 4. 3g

Ingredients:

- 1 1/2 cups+ 2 tbsps pure date sugar
- 4 medium banana, peeled and sliced
- 2 cups unsweetened almond milk
- 1/2 tsp salt
- 6 tbsps corn-starch
- 4 tbsps cold plant butter, cut into 4 pieces
- 4 cups cashew cream
- 2 tsps vanilla extract

Procedure:

1. Take a medium pot, mix the almond milk, cashew cream, date sugar, and salt.
2. Now, cook over medium heat until slightly thickened, 10 to 15 minutes.
3. Then, stir in the corn-starch, plant butter, vanilla extract, and banana extract.
4. Now, cook further for 1 to 2 minutes or until the pudding thickens.
5. Dish the pudding into 4 serving bowls and chill in the refrigerator for at least 1 hour.
6. To serve, top with the bananas and enjoy!

Servings: 8

Preparation Time: 15-30 minutes

Per Serving: Calories 882 Fats 66. 35g Carbs 64. 5g Protein 19. 95g

Ingredients:

- 4 cups fresh cranberries
- 2 tsps vanilla extract
- 4 tbsps pure date syrup
- 4 tbsps pure date sugar
- 32 oz. cashew cream
- 8 tbsps plant butter
- 6 tbsps unsweetened cocoa powder

Procedure:

1. Set a silicone egg tray aside.
2. Puree the cranberries, date syrup, and vanilla in a blender until smooth.
3. Now, add the cashew cream and plant butter to a medium pot.
4. Heat over medium heat until the mixture is well combined.
5. Then, turn the heat off.
6. Now, mix in the cranberry mixture and divide the mixture into the muffin holes.
7. Refrigerate for 40 minutes or until firm.

8. After, remove the tray and pop out the truffles.
9. Meanwhile, mix the cocoa powder and date sugar on a plate.
10. In the end, roll the truffles in the mixture until well dusted and serve.

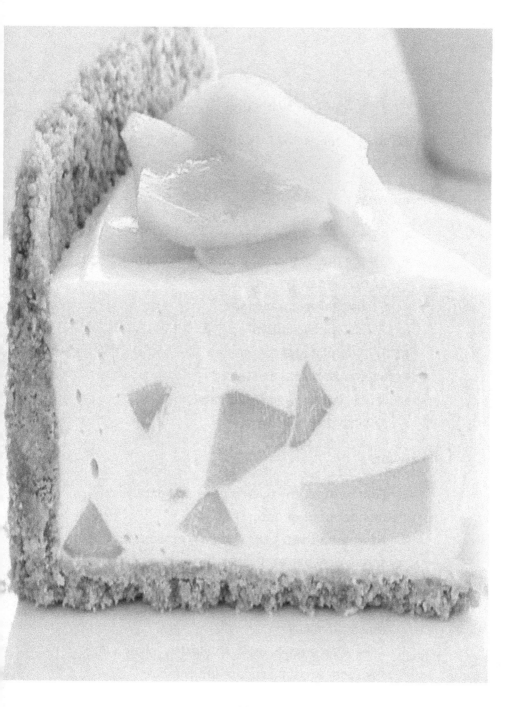

Servings: 8

Preparation Time: 15-30 minutes

Per Serving: Calories 337 Fats 28g Carbs 21. 3g Protein 5. 4g

Ingredients:

- 6 tbsps pure date sugar
- 2 large ripe mangoes, peeled and chopped
- 12 oz. cashew cream cheese
- 6 tsps agar-agar powder
- 1/2 cup of coconut milk
- 1/2 cup plant butter, melted
- 2 lemons, zested and juiced
- 1 1/3 cups toasted rolled oats
- 1/2 cup just-boiled water

Procedure:

1. First, process the oats, butter, and date sugar in a blender until smooth.
2. Now, pour the mixture into a greased 9-inch springform pan and press the mixture onto the bottom of the pan.
3. Refrigerate for 30 minutes until firm while you make the filling.
4. Take a large bowl, using an electric mixer, whisk the cashew cream cheese until smooth.

5. Beat in coconut milk, lemon zest, and lemon juice.
6. Now, mix the boiled water and agar-agar powder until dissolved and whisk this mixture into the creamy mix. Fold in the mangoes.
7. Then, remove the cake pan from the fridge and pour in the mango mixture.
8. Shake the pan to ensure smooth layering on top.
9. Refrigerate further for at least 3 hours.
10. In the end, remove the cheesecake from the fridge, release the cake pan, slice, and serve.

Servings: 8

Preparation Time: 15-30 minutes

Per Serving: Calories 354 Fats 26. 7g Carbs 27. 7g Protein 6. 4g

Ingredients:

- 6 tbsps pure date sugar
- 12 oz. cashew cream cheese
- 1/2 cup oats milk
- 1 1/3 cups toasted rolled oats
- 4 tbsps toasted cashew nuts, chopped
- 1/2 cup plant butter, melted
- 1/2 cup just-boiled water
- 6 tsps agar-agar powder
- 8 plums, cored and finely diced

Procedure:

1. First, process the oats, butter, and date sugar in a blender until smooth.
2. Now, pour the mixture into a greased 9-inch springform pan and press the mixture onto the bottom of the pan.
3. Refrigerate for 30 minutes until firm while you make the filling.

4. Take a large bowl, using an electric mixer, whisk the cashew cream cheese until smooth. Beat in the oats milk.
5. Now, mix the boiled water and agar-agar powder until dissolved and whisk this mixture into the creamy mix.
6. Then, fold in the plums.
7. After, remove the cake pan from the fridge and pour in the plum mixture.
8. Shake the pan to ensure smooth layering on top.
9. Refrigerate further for at least 3 hours.
10. Take out the cake pan, release the cake, and garnish with the cashew nuts.
11. Finally, slice and serve.

Servings: 40

Preparation Time: 25 minutes

Per Serving: Calories: 101; Fat: 2.5g; Carbs: 17.2g; Protein: 2.8g

Ingredients:

- 2 teaspoons baking soda
- 3 cups rolled oats
- A pinch of grated nutmeg
- A pinch of coarse salt
- 1 cup brown sugar
- 1 teaspoon cinnamon
- 1 cup dried cranberries
- 1 1/3 cups peanut butter
- 2 teaspoons vanilla extract
- 2 medium bananas, mashed
- 2/3 cup oat milk

Procedure:

1. Begin by preheating your oven to 350 degrees F.
2. Take a mixing bowl, thoroughly combine the dry ingredients.
3. Take another bowl, combine the wet ingredients.
4. Then, stir the wet mixture into the dry ingredients; mix to combine well.

5. Now, spread the batter mixture in a parchment-lined baking pan.
6. Bake in the preheated oven for about 20 minutes.
7. Then, let it cool on a wire rack. Cut into squares and enjoy!

Servings: 8

Preparation Time: 2 hours

Per Serving: Calories: 377; Fat: 6.5g; Carbs: 72g; Protein: 10.7g

Ingredients:

- 20 ounces day-old bread, cut into cubes
- 4 cups coconut milk
- 1 cup coconut sugar
- 2 teaspoons vanilla extract
- 1 teaspoon ground cloves
- 1 teaspoon ground cinnamon
- 1 cup Sultanas

Procedure:

1. First, place the bread cubes in a lightly oiled baking dish.
2. Now, blend the milk, sugar, vanilla, ground cloves, and cinnamon until creamy and smooth.
3. Then, spoon the mixture all over the bread cubes, pressing them with a wide spatula to soak well; fold in Sultanas and set aside for about 1 hour.
4. Now, bake in the preheated oven at 350 degrees F for about 1 hour or until the top of your pudding is golden brown.

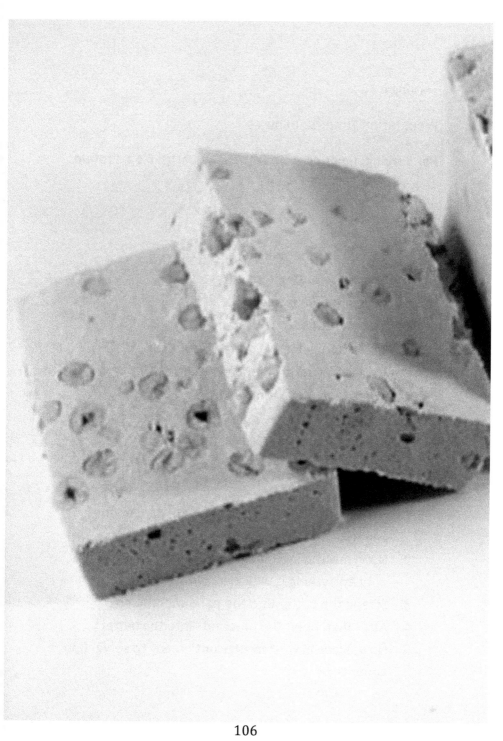

Servings: 32

Preparation Time: 10 minutes

Per Serving: Calories: 169; Fat: 15.5g; Carbs: 6.6g; Protein: 1.9g

Ingredients:

- 1/2 cup coconut oil, melted
- 1 cup hazelnuts, chopped
- 1 cup almond butter
- 8 tablespoons agave nectar
- 1/4 teaspoon freshly grated nutmeg
- 1 teaspoon pure almond extract
- 1 teaspoon pure vanilla extract
- 1 cup tahini
- 1/4 teaspoon salt

Procedure:

1. First, line a square baking pan with parchment paper.
2. Now, mix the ingredients, except for the hazelnuts, until everything is well incorporated.
3. Scrape the batter into the parchment-lined pan.
4. After that, press the hazelnuts into the batter.
5. Now, place in your freezer until ready to serve. Bon appétit!

Servings: 24

Preparation Time: 10 minutes + chilling time

Per Serving: Calories: 226; Fat: 15.9g; Carbs: 19.8g; Protein: 5.1g

Ingredients:

Crust:

- 2 cups fresh dates, pitted
- 2 cups raw almonds

Topping:

- 1 cup dates, pitted
- 2 cups raw cashew nuts, soaked overnight and drained
- 2 oranges, freshly squeezed
- 1 cup raw sunflower seeds, soaked overnight, and drained
- 1/2 cup coconut oil, softened

Garnish:

- 4 tablespoons caramel topping

Procedure:

1. Take your food processor, blend the crust ingredients until the mixture comes together; press the crust into a lightly greased muffin tin.
2. Then, blend the topping ingredients until creamy and smooth.
3. Now, spoon the topping mixture onto the crust, creating a flat surface with a spatula.
4. Place these mini cheesecakes in your freezer for about 3 hours.
5. Then, garnish with caramel topping. Bon appétit!

Lightning Source UK Ltd.
Milton Keynes UK
UKHW021821160421
382091UK00005B/70

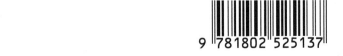